Anti-Inflammatory Diet

*The Best Recipes to Relieve Pain,
Fight Inflammation and Restore Health*

© Copyright 2016 by LR Books - All rights reserved.

This document is geared towards providing exact and reliable information in regards to the topic and issue covered. The publication is sold with the idea that the publisher is not required to render accounting, officially permitted, or otherwise, qualified services. If advice is necessary, legal or professional, a practiced individual in the profession should be ordered.

- From a Declaration of Principles which was accepted and approved equally by a Committee of the American Bar Association and a Committee of Publishers and Associations.

In no way is it legal to reproduce, duplicate, or transmit any part of this document in either electronic means or in printed format. Recording of this publication is strictly prohibited and any storage of this document is not allowed unless with written permission from the publisher. All rights reserved.

The information provided herein is stated to be truthful and consistent, in that any liability, in terms of inattention or otherwise, by any usage or abuse of any policies, processes, or directions contained within is the solitary and utter responsibility of the recipient reader. Under no circumstances will any legal responsibility or blame be held against the publisher for any reparation, damages, or monetary loss due to the information herein, either directly or indirectly.

Respective authors own all copyrights not held by the publisher.

The information herein is offered for informational purposes solely, and is universal as so. The presentation of the information is without contract or any type of guarantee assurance.

The trademarks that are used are without any consent, and the publication of the trademark is without permission or backing by the trademark owner. All trademarks and brands within this book are for clarifying purposes only and are the owned by the owners themselves, not affiliated with this document.

TABLE OF CONTENTS

INTRODUCTION 1

CHAPTER 1: A Different View on Inflammation 7

CHAPTER 2: Food Items That Have Anti-Inflammatory Power 12

CHAPTER 3: Planning an Anti-Inflammatory Diet 23

CHAPTER 4: Anti-Inflammatory Breakfast Recipes 25

CHAPTER 5: Anti-Inflammatory Soups 31

CHAPTER 6: Lunch or Dinner Recipes 39

CHAPTER 7: Smoothies and Teas 46

CHAPTER 8: Eat an Anti-Inflammatory Diet in Real Practice 50

CHAPTER 9: This Diet Can Still be Beneficial Even if Inflammation is Not a Problem 56

CONCLUSION   60

Introduction

I want to thank you and congratulate you for downloading the book, *"Anti-Inflammatory Diet: The Best Recipes to Relieve Pain, Fight Inflammation and Restore Health."*

This book contains proven steps and strategies on how to reduce inflammation with the foods that you commonly use in your kitchen.

Our body is one of the most incredible machines the world has ever seen. Uniquely designed to be the ultimate in recycling, it can restore itself whenever it is faced with physical harm. Just as man-made machinery will all eventually break down and need repair, human bodies will also suffer from the wear and tear of life, and will eventually need fixing. The difference however, is that under the right conditions, the body can and will do all of this itself. One of the ways this can happen is through the natural process of inflammation, a primary tool of our own immune system.

Inflammation is the body's way of initiating the self-repair of damaged tissue or ridding the system of harmful toxins that may have accumulated over time. There are many reasons why the body might develop inflammation; it could be the result of something small like an insect bite or something as serious as an infection that has invaded the body. Whatever the case, it is through this reaction that the body gets what it needs to heal itself. This could mean more blood supplied to the affected area as a means of eliminating the toxins that are causing harm or it could mean sending more white blood cells to the area to start healing damaged tissue.

In most cases, the inflammation occurs naturally in response to a condition that has damaged the body in some way. It is an automatic defense mechanism that protects us from illness or injury and its primary role is to localize or even eliminate the source or the cause of harm. While it may be a cause of discomfort and even pain, without it self-healing can be much more difficult and it can take much longer to recover.

In a healthy individual this discomfort could last only a few days and, as the healing process progresses, the condition will gradually fade. This is called acute inflammation and is perfectly normal. However, there are cases where the inflammation tends to linger in the body for an extended period of time, lasting for days, weeks, or even months on end. This is referred to as chronic inflammation and can lead to a wide range of complications that could be even more harmful to your health.

How It Works

When an area of the body is injured or infected, the brain receives a signal that causes it to release several chemicals (bradykinin, histamine, and prostaglandins) that are immediately sent to the affected area. These chemicals form a line of defense that accomplishes two things. First, it will cause the area to swell, blocking the infection from advancing to other nearby cells that are unharmed and second, it will send a message to the brain that more white blood cells are needed at the site to start the repair work. In the case of physical trauma, the inflammation stops or reduces the spread of injury to the surrounding cells and tissues. With the redness, heat, pain, and swelling that result, it creates a better environment for faster healing.

The white blood cells will feed on any germs or toxins and then gradually die off when they are no longer needed. What's left will collect in the form of pus, which will eventually be expelled through natural bodily functions.

Ideally, this condition works well and in most cases, once the body heals the inflammation will go away on its own. But, there are times when the body's system gets out of whack and you can end up with too much swelling or a prolonged condition, which can impair your ability to function under normal circumstances. Cases of asthma and bronchitis are probably two of the most common incidences of chronic inflammation that if left untreated could become life threatening.

Does this mean that inflammation is bad and should be avoided at all costs? Ironically, the answer is no. The reality is that inflammation is not usually the problem. It's a natural bodily reaction and an indicator that something is wrong and needs to be fixed. However, just because inflammation is not always bad, it does not mean that it should go untreated. In the case of chronic inflammation, it can lead to other problems with your health.

When you have chronic inflammation, the brain is continuously receiving signals to send more helper cells to the affected area. This keeps the immune system constantly working under pressure, which will make it less efficient in protecting the body when it needs help the most. The result could be an excess of swelling and scar tissue build up, which can have a major impact on the body's ability to function normally.

Cases of asthma and bronchitis are perfect examples of this. When unwelcome toxins invade the airways they build up in the passageways to the lungs, making it difficult to breath. While it may feel like congestion, it is inflammation that is closing up the airways. It is easy to see why this condition could quickly turn into a life threatening situation if not treated properly.

Why Food Matters

Unlike other organs in the body, the immune system is "a system," which means that it is not one single entity, like the liver or the heart muscle, that is setting up a line of defense for the entire body, but a collection of signals and reactions that communicate and respond to one another to protect the body from external influences and invaders. Think of it like an army of troops sent to protect the borders of a country from unwanted attack. There is not usually one line of defense but several, and some lines where the security has been breached will be more heavily reinforced where others will not.

In the body, the gastrointestinal (GI) tract is one of those defense lines. Your GI tract contains 150 times more surface area than your external skin and makes up approximately 80% of your entire immune system. This is because your digestive tract is more likely to be exposed to harmful toxins and bacterial invasions than any other body part. When you consider that the average person will consume over 25 tons of food during the course of their lifetime, you can see why your digestive system needs to be finely tuned to protect your health. It must determine which foods you consume contain harmful toxins and try to eliminate them, but at the same time serve as a gateway for letting in essential nutrients that can be used to fuel your body and allow it to survive.

The GI Tract or GALT (gut associated lymphoid tissue) is a group or a layer of specialized cells that work together to perform certain functions. These tissues include the tonsils, Peyer's patches, lamina propria of the GI tract and the appendix. Together these tissues hold the key responsibility of keeping a vigilant watch over your immune system and protecting it from harmful invaders.

This means that to protect the body from excessive inflammation, the line of defense should logically start with the diet. By choosing the right foods to eat you can either support your immune system or damage it further.

This book contains proven steps and strategies on how to reduce inflammation with the foods that you commonly use in your kitchen. Hopefully it will serve as a catalyst for you to change the types of foods you eat to help avoid inflammation or at least reduce it. It provides you with a list of anti-inflammatory foods to keep in your arsenal to help you in your fight. With better food choices, you'll be able to improve the overall health of your digestive tract and the overall health of your GALT too.

Just keep in mind that this is not a one-time process. Eating a healthy food once won't help you to increase your immunity and/or reduce inflammation. It won't be an instant fix either. This means to improve your system and reduce the inflammation in your body, it will require making healthy eating a habit. So, let's begin this healthy journey together, and learn more about the anti-inflammatory diet.

CHAPTER 1

A Different View on Inflammation

Let us begin by learning about the six main causes of inflammation. This will help us to see when inflammation is good for us and when it becomes a danger to our health.

The first cause of inflammation in the body comes from toxic elements getting into the system. These can range from simple toxins that come from things like consuming alcohol or more complex ones found in many common drugs. Whenever you consume any irritant in either the chemical or physical form, it will cause inflammation as the body tries to rid itself of the irritant and start the healing process.

The second cause is from infections. This is usually brought about by a pathogenic element such as a virus or bacteria, yeast, fungus, or other parasite entering the body; all of which can introduce infections into your system. When these parasites attack, the immune system will fight back and the first sign will be inflammation.

The third cause can be from allergies. If you are allergic to any food (natural or synthetic), your body will protect itself by producing inflammation in the form of an allergic reaction. This is not a healing process in itself but if you leave the inflammation unchecked, it could trigger an autoimmune disease, which can open up a host of other more serious medical problems.

The fourth cause of inflammation comes when a nutritional imbalance occurs, which can trigger a hormonal disturbance. This imbalance is not limited to some type of deficiency in the physical make-up of the body but can also be the result of an excessive intake of certain nutrients. Those who overindulge in certain foods and drinks may be opening themselves up to more inflammation as the body tries to rid itself of the excess. Remember, too much of a good thing may not always be good for you.

The fifth and sixth causes can be triggered by trauma. When the body experiences physical trauma, inflammation is triggered to prevent the injury from spreading to other parts of the body. It can also force the body to protect your inner organs from further damage. And emotional trauma increases the cortisol and adrenaline levels in the body, which also cause inflammation.

All of these causes are the result of an invasion or an infiltration of unwanted or harmful substances entering the body. In these cases, inflammation can be a very good thing. But our concern in this book stems from what to do about inflammation when it gets out of control.

Whenever your body experiences these typical triggers, it will cause inflammation as a means of self-preservation. When it occurs for the right reason, it will attack the pathogens or other invaders protecting you and preventing further harm. Keep in mind that the brain will provide more protector cells to the site of inflammation for as long as it is needed. But if the immune system is out of balance or is not functioning properly, it will end up functioning on overdrive all the time. This can lead to more damage, especially if there is no pathogen or invader for it to fight.

When the infection is counter-attacked, the immune system will communicate it to the brain by means of natural chemicals, which will reduce the inflammation. However, in certain cases where people have high C-reactive proteins (the substance produced by the liver that increases when inflammation develops in the body), the body could remain in the defensive mode, even after the pathogens have been destroyed. This is because the counter signal sent by the immune system to the brain is never received.

Acute and Chronic Inflammation

It is also important that you know the difference between good and bad inflammation. This will help you to determine when you need to be concerned and when things are proceeding as they should.

Injuries and small infections will automatically trigger inflammation. You should expect to experience pain, redness, swelling, and heat in the affected area. It could be present for a few days or only a few minutes, before it begins to disappear. This is called acute inflammation. In most of these cases, the problem of acute inflammation will naturally be resolved on its own without any additional assistance.

When the inflammation is caused by any pathogen that is non-degradable (viruses, foreign bodies, auto-immune reactions, or other similar invaders), the swelling could remain for several months or even for years. Over time, this can destroy surrounding tissue causing excessive scarring. This is called chronic inflammation.

Whether it is acute or chronic inflammation, it is important to improve the health of our immune system to ensure that the problem is reduced as soon as possible. There are a lot of drugs on the market today that can help with the healing process. But you run the risk of side effects causing even more severe problems with additional harm to the body. This is where you can make better use of the anti-inflammatory diet. As you read on in this book, you'll learn more specifics about the anti-inflammatory diet.

CHAPTER 2

Food Items That Have Anti-Inflammatory Power

There are a lot of foods that can help you to reduce the symptoms and the effects of inflammation in the body. You might already be consuming a lot of them without knowing their true value. This chapter is dedicated to giving you a detailed list of many of the foods you can consume to fight off inflammation and give you a healthy body in return.

Proteins

You'll need foods high in protein to boost the immune system. Numerous research studies have shown that diets low in protein can result in a significant depletion of the immune cells. It can also render the system unable to produce needed antibodies or cope with other immune-related problems. With even a 25% reduction in necessary protein, the entire immune system could be negatively compromised.

Proteins are comprised of the 20 amino acids the body needs to repair itself. They are essential for the immune system to work properly. Any diet that gives support to a healthy immune system should include foods high in protein like eggs, fish, and shellfish. There are also many vegetables and grains that can also be a good source of protein.

Essential Vitamins

You'll also need to stock up on foods that are rich in essential vitamins to boost your immune system. Nearly every vitamin found in food sources can help build a healthy immune system but there are some vitamins that are more effective than others.

These include Vitamins C, B5, B6, Folic Acid, Thiamin, Riboflavin, and Vitamin B12.

Vitamin C is considered an immune stimulant; in fact, it ranks at the top of the list. When you have an adequate supply of vitamin C it can reduce the amount of time and the severity of the symptoms you experience as a result of respiratory infections; it can also promote phagocytic cell function, and healthy T-cell function. Also because it is also an antioxidant it can help to reduce inflammation while healing.

Vitamin C can be found in citrus fruits and many vegetables including asparagus, beet greens, bokchoy, broccoli, collard greens, kale, mustard greens, swiss chard, and turnip greens.

B Vitamins are also essential for boosting the immune system. B5 for example, encourages the promotion, production, and the release of antibodies.

Folic Acid can increase the number of T-cells and improve effectiveness of the soluble factors in the body.

Thiamin and Riboflavin can enhance normal antibody response.

Vitamin B12 can boost phagocytic cells and even improve T-cell functions.

These vitamins can be found in almost all whole grains, vegetables, and fruits, which can be excellent sources to add to your regular diet. Some vegetables however, are better sources than others. For example, Romaine lettuce contains a lot of B1, B2, C, and Folate. Turnip greens and spinach contain high levels of folate, B6, and C. Cauliflower has high amounts of vitamin C, and B6, and Crimini mushrooms contain a lot of B2. By having a good mix of these vegetables in your diet, you can be assured that your immune system will have as much help as it can get.

Minerals support your immune system and a healthy dose of minerals will keep it functioning properly. Zinc for example, is considered to be an immune-stimulant that can boost T-cell function.

There are many other minerals that can make for a healthy immune system. Most people are aware of what happens in the body when there's an iron deficiency. It results in impaired responses and defective cell function. Copper deficiencies can produce impaired development of cells and a lack of selenium and manganese can interfere with the healing process in the body.

Excellent sources for these minerals are found in seeds, nuts, beans, mushrooms, greens, asparagus, and squash.

Antioxidants encourage the immune system function. Reactive oxygen species, free radicals, and other harmful molecules build up at the site of an infection. The body needs these to help kill damaged and unhealthy cells. Antioxidants help the immune system by disarming the harmful molecules after they have completed their job in preventing the damage from spreading to other parts of the body.

Good sources of antioxidants can be found in foods like carrots, cherries, strawberries and tomatoes.

Of course, this is not a complete list of essential foods you can have in your diet, but it can serve as a guide to help you to decide which foods to eat to boost your immune system. Below is a list of essential foods that you'll need to keep in stock to support your anti-inflammatory diet.

Fatty Fish

These could include salmon, sardines, tuna, mackerel, and any fish rich in omega-3 fatty acids. Incorporate these into your diet several times a week.

Whole Grains

It is important to know the difference between whole grains and refined grains. Cereal, rice, white bread, and other similar grains are made from refined grains, which offer minimal nutritional value for the body. Whole grains have essential fiber and can help you to reduce inflammation by controlling the level of C-reactive protein in your body.

Dark Leafy Vegetables

Vegetables like kale, spinach, swiss chard, and collard greens are some of the leafy vegetables, which can increase flavonoids and vitamin C in the body. This will help to reduce the cellular damage and increase the speed of reducing inflammation in the body. Instead of adding these leaves to your meals as an additional vegetable, it is better to incorporate them as juices or smoothies and have them the first thing in the morning when you wake up. If you plan to use this method, remember to drink a lot of water to aid in the digestion process.

Nuts

All healthy nuts (unsalted and baked) will provide you with omega-3 fatty acids. The best and most beneficial nuts to include in your diet are almonds. By incorporating nuts into your meals and snacks, you may see a significant reduction in inflammation in as little as six weeks. Caution is warranted though. Nuts are a powerhouse of goodness but are also a source of concentrated calories. Munching on a handful with coffee is definitely an improvement on a sugary pastry but, if you are watching your weight, be wary of consuming too many.

Soy

All soy products work to reduce the negative effects of inflammation in the heart and bones. Try to find naturally produced soy and avoid Genetically Modified as it may cause additional problems to your health overall.

Peppers

Both bell peppers and hot peppers contain capsaicin. This is the chemical that is used in many topical creams that are used to treat inflammation. Adding a lot of peppers to your diet can reduce the pain of inflammation.

Tomatoes

This one can be a little tricky. Tomatoes can help to reduce the inflammation in many parts of the body for certain people. But this may not work for everyone in the same way. If it works for you, it is best to have cooked tomatoes rather than raw. This is because when cooked, tomatoes have a higher amount of lycopene, which can reduce the amount of inflammation that you experience.

Beets

All kinds of beets can reduce inflammation and protect the body from heart disease and certain types of cancer.

Berries

Blueberries and raspberries are known to have antioxidant properties. This can be especially helpful with problems with intestinal inflammation.

Onions

Onions have a pain killing property. They will reduce the pain caused by inflammation and also reduce the effects of inflammation on other organs in the body.

Olive Oil

Another similar painkiller is olive oil, which acts in much the same way as the onion.

Tart Cherries

These have a higher anti-inflammatory content than any other food product. It helps to reduce the inflammation in blood vessels and also reduces the pain due to inflammation in other tissues and organs. It is better to incorporate it into the diet as a juice.

Shitake Mushrooms

This mushroom has the natural ability to reduce and even inhibit the amount of inflammation that may occur in the body.

Spices That Fight Inflammation

There are four significant spices that are known to reduce inflammation:

    Ginger

    Cloves

    Rosemary

    Turmeric

These have a very high anti-inflammatory effect, and also help to reverse the damage done by inflammation to some extent. The other spices known to have potent anti-inflammatory power are:

Cinnamon

Oregano

Marjoram

Thyme

Sage

Black Pepper

This is not the complete list of all the food items that have high levels of anti-inflammatory effects. Other foods that can be used to fight inflammation are:

Green tea

Cannabis

Basil leaves

Grapple plan or wood spider or devil's claw

Hyssop (great for lung inflammation)

Jamaican ginger

Apricot, Avocado, Cantaloupe, Grapefruit, Papaya, Lemon, Pineapple

Asparagus, Broccoli, Bok Choy

Carrot, Cauliflower, Cucumber, Pumpkin

Dark Chocolate

Eggs

Flaxseeds, Fennel

Defining Your Enemy in the Food Pyramid

Eating right also means that you should remove the toxic foods from your regular diet. It is important to note that a toxic food need not be a poisonous one. For certain people, there are some foods that will increase the inflammation or the pain caused by it. So, if you're sensitive to any of these foods, you should take extra precautions and try to avoid them as much as possible.

Red meat

Processed food – canned fruits and vegetables are considered to be processed foods

Common cooking oil

Dairy products

Trans fats found in fried foods, peanut butter, margarine, and others

Alcohol

Any kind of food additives such as preservatives, flavor enhancers, and others

Sugar in any form other than natural fruit

Certain food items that can cause inflammation when you consume them. The most common examples are coffee, cheese, and chocolate, but there are many others.

Now, that you have lists of foods that you should consume or avoid, you're ready to start working on planning your anti-inflammatory diet.

CHAPTER 3

Planning an Anti-Inflammatory Diet

Planning an anti-inflammatory diet involves much more than getting a few recipes together. The diet focuses on having a variety of food items to keep the diet interesting. You can include as much and as many fresh foods as you want unless you are allergic to them.

You need to reduce or eliminate your consumption of fast foods as well as any processed foods you consume. It's essential to make sure that you stay hydrated; that means drinking a lot of water to help the body expel the waste. It should be plain water without any additives like cordial or coffee. You can have water with a little lemon juice, mix it with fruit juice, or as an unsweetened tea.

It is also important to make sure that you consume 2,000 to 3,000 calories a day if you're an adult. And no more than 50% of the calories should come from carbohydrates, 30% should come from fat, and the remaining from protein. But make sure that the meals are balanced, do not dedicate one meal to carbohydrates, another for fat, and another for something else. Instead, make sure that all the elements of the diet are included in every single meal.

Your carbohydrates should be consumed in the form of low glycemic food. Low glycemic foods are those that do not increase your blood sugar levels. Barley, quinoa, sweet corn, lentils, yogurt, soy milk, beans, chickpeas, almost all fruits, prunes, and many others are all considered to be low glycemic foods. However, beans, squashes, whole grains, and others should be included more often than the others.

Fats should be mostly monounsaturated. Saturated fats like chicken skin, cheese, cream, butter, and other similar foods should be avoided. If you have an autoimmune disorder or any problems related to kidney or liver, avoid consuming an abundance of protein. Alternatively, when you do consume protein, try to get it in the vegetable form rather than from animal sources.

Also for fiber, it is better to opt for vegetables and berries than cereals.

CHAPTER 4

Anti-Inflammatory Breakfast Recipes

When you get right down to it, most Americans consume far too much of omega-6 fatty acids and far too little of the omega-3. While we need to have them both to survive, making sure that you have a healthy balance between the two is essential. When planning your anti-inflammatory breakfasts focus on using healthy, unprocessed foods so that you can keep the amount of fat you consume under control. With fewer fats in your body you can limit the amount of inflammation you will get.

1. Banana Coconut Smoothie

½ cup of coconut milk

½ cup of almond milk

1 banana

1 handful of flax seeds

Cinnamon

Mix all the ingredients together in a blender and blend until smooth. This is a quick and healthy, low fat breakfast that can get your body going and still offer you the ability to lower the amount of inflammation in your body.

2. Fruit and Yogurt

Chop up your favorite fresh fruit and mix with a cup of Greek or plain yogurt. You can enhance the flavor by adding a handful of nuts to add more texture. Make sure that you avoid the fruit flavored yogurts that are offered in your local supermarket. It is not the same and may contain lots of harmful additives that you don't need. If at all possible, it is best to get home-made or organically prepared yogurt whenever possible.

3. Yogurt Cereal

You can take any whole grain cereal and mix in pomegranate seeds and greek yogurt. It boosts the flavor and is full of all the essential ingredients you need to fight inflammation.

4. Rice Bread with Apricots

Take dried apricots, greek yogurt, and honey and mix together in a bowl. Use rice bread as a filler to add a little substance to the meal.

5. Oatmeal

Cooked oatmeal is an excellent breakfast food for all sorts of reasons. While the taste may be bland, you can flavor it up with all kind of nuts, berries, and fruits, which will add enough sweetness to satisfy your sweet tooth when you need it.

6. Spinach and Mushroom Omelet

Finely chop ¼ cup each of spinach and mushrooms. Beat two eggs together and add a dash of cayenne powder along with the chopped ingredients. Make an omelet and serve with a slice of whole grain bread.

7. Pancakes with Berries

Mix together 1 cup of Buckwheat flour with 2 Tablespoons of Tapioca flour. Add two eggs and blend together to make a pancake batter. Add in enough plain yogurt to make the mixture pourable. Mix in your favorite berries and cook the pancakes until golden.

8. Ginger Oatmeal

Mix a half a cup of oats in one cup of water. Add one teaspoon of ground ginger and a quarter teaspoon each of cinnamon and nutmeg. Mix in ¼ cup of cranberries or any other berry you like. Bring the whole mixture to a boil. Add in a handful of flaxseed and let it simmer for five minutes. If you use steel cut oats, it will take longer to cook through.

If you prefer a heavier breakfast to start the day, try some of these recipes for a meal that will stick to your ribs for a little longer.

9. Pork and Eggs

This is a nice substitute for the traditional bacon and eggs breakfast. Instead of the greasy bacon try using apple pork instead.

- 2 oz. center cut pork loin chop
- 1 ½ tsp. of olive oil
- 1 apple slice
- 1/3 teaspoon of cinnamon
- ½ cup of egg whites

Lightly cook the pork in olive oil over medium-high heat and brown it on all sides.

In a separate pan, sauté the apples and cinnamon together until the apples are just barely tender. Place the pork and apples on a plate and add a couple of scrambled egg whites to complete the dish.

10. Baked Eggs with Vegetables

 6 Roma tomatoes, chopped into small chunks

 1 Tablespoon of salt

 1 teaspoon of olive oil

 2 Tablespoons of vegetable stock

 ½ cup of onions, chopped fine

 ½ cup of chopped ham

 1 cup of chopped spinach

 1 ¼ cup of egg whites

 ¼ cup of cream cheese Tofutti

 ¼ cup of fresh chives, chopped

 3 Tablespoons of unsweetened almond milk

 1 orange

First preheat the oven to 350F. Boil a small kettle of water and coat two oven safe bowls with olive oil. Use spray if you prefer and then set them aside. In a separate bowl toss the peeled and chopped tomatoes in the salt and then spoon them evenly in the oiled bowls.

In a large skillet, mix together the oil, stock, and onions and then cook in skillet over medium to high heat. Make sure that you stir them occasionally to keep them from sticking. Cook until translucent, which should take about 4 minutes. Add in the ham and continue cooking for an additional minute. Remove the pan from heat and add in the spinach and toss the mixture together until the greens just start to wilt.

In a separate bowl whisk the egg whites, Tofutti, chives, and the almond milk together. Divide the mixture evenly between the two bowls and mix well with the tomatoes and add in the ham and vegetables.

Place both bowls on a baking pan and put on the middle oven rack. Fill a baking pan with the boiling water up to the halfway mark on the sides and place in the bottom of the oven. Bake the quiche for 25-30 minutes and carefully remove from the oven, season with salt and pepper to taste and serve with orange slices.

CHAPTER 5

Anti-Inflammatory Soups

Soups are a great meal that can be prepared ahead of time. They work well if you're like most people and have a pretty busy schedule. They can be frozen and kept for quite a while and simply reheated when you're ready to eat. They're also versatile and are suitable for lunch or dinner, especially when the weather starts to turn cold and you want something that can really warm up your insides. Soups also have a soothing effect when you're dealing with viral infections and respiratory problems. Here is a selection of anti-inflammatory soups you can make ahead of time and have on hand when you need them.

1. Celery Soup

1 bunch of celery

4 onions

1 medium sized leek

1 medium potato

Chicken pieces

Yogurt

Parsley

Chop the celery, onions, and leek and mix together. Place in a pot of water and bring to a boil. Peel and chop the potato and add to the boiling mixture. Cook until the potato becomes tender. (If you are not a vegan, you can add chicken pieces at the same time as the potato.) When cooked through, allow it to cool before adding the yogurt and chopped parsley to finish it off.

2. Leek Soup

2 medium leeks

1 bunch of parsley

4 large green onions

1 zucchini

Boil leeks and parsley stems for five minutes. Add chopped green onions and zucchini, and add more water. Boil until they become soft and can be smashed with the back of a spoon.

3. Cold Cucumber Soup

6 medium cucumbers

½ cup of chopped parsley

lemon juice

1½ cups of half-and-half

1 cup of yogurt

Salt

Blend the cucumber, parsley, and lemon juice in a blender. Add in the half-and-half, yogurt, and salt. Refrigerate and chill before serving.

4. Pumpkin Soup

1 cup of chopped onions

1 clove of garlic

1 inch of minced ginger

5½ cup of vegetable stock

4 cups of pumpkin puree

Salt

Thyme

In a pot, add onion, garlic, ginger, and ½ cup of vegetable stock. Cook together for about five minutes. Add in the pumpkin puree, salt, thyme, and the remaining five cups of stock. Cook for an additional 30 minutes. Use a blender to make it smooth and serve with chopped parsley.

5. Gazpacho

Most people don't think of soup when it comes to warm weather but a cold gazpacho can not only boost your immune system it is also an anti-fungal and anti-bacterial dish that is one of the most nutritious meals you can find. Add in a cup of coconut milk and go heavy on the garlic and this becomes a power soup that can do wonders for your health.

1 minced onion

1 teaspoon of coconut oil

1 teaspoon of turmeric

1 teaspoon of ginger

1 teaspoon of mustard powder

1 teaspoon of curry powder

½ teaspoon of cinnamon

½ teaspoon cayenne

1 cup of lentils

1 ½ cups of vegetable broth

1 ½ cups of coconut milk (unsweetened)

3 cloves of minced garlic (let sit for 15 minutes or more before cooking)

¼ cup of yogurt

In a medium saucepan, sauté the onions in the coconut oil over medium heat until they become translucent. Mix in the spices and continue to cook for an additional 3 minutes or until the aroma of the ingredients becomes quite strong. Add in the lentils, vegetable broth and the coconut milk. Bring the entire mixture to a boil and then reduce heat and let simmer uncovered for up to 45 minutes. When the lentils are soft and have absorbed the majority of the liquid, turn off the heat, add in the garlic and stir it together. Mix until the garlic starts to cook from the heat of the soup. Chill before serving. Swirl in coconut milk or yogurt before serving.

6. Carrot and Ginger Soup

1 Tablespoon coconut oil

1 chopped medium brown onion

2 cloves of minced garlic

2 cm pieces of fresh ginger

2 cm pieces of fresh galangal

1 cm of fresh turmeric

1 diced red chili

1 ½ lbs. of carrots, washed, peeled, and chopped

2 cups of chicken or vegetable stock

2 cups of water

5 cm of lemongrass stalks

In a saucepan, heat the coconut oil over medium-high heat. Add the onion and sauté until soft and tender. Stir in the garlic, ginger, galangal, turmeric, and chili and cook for an additional 5 minutes. Add the carrots, stock and lemongrass and bring the entire mixture to a boil. Lower the heat and allow to simmer for up to 20 minutes or until the carrots are softened. Remove the lemongrass and discard. Blend the soup in a blender until the texture is smooth. Serve with a drizzle of yogurt and hot chili sauce.

7. Vegetable Soup

2 Tablespoons of olive oil

1 diced carrot

1 stalk diced celery

1 finely chopped red onion

3 cloves of minced garlic

1 diced red bell pepper

2 cups of shredded cabbage

½ cup of green lentils

1 teaspoon of dried oregano

1 strip of kombu

3 cups of vegetable stock

Anti-Inflammatory Diet

2 cups of finely chopped kale

½ bunch of chopped parsley

1 cup of cooked brown rice

1 teaspoon of Basil pesto

Heat the oil in a large stockpot. Add in the carrot, celery, onion, garlic, and the red bell pepper. Sauté thoroughly until vegetables are tender. This should take about 5 minutes. Mix in the cabbage and cook for an additional 5 minutes. Add in the lentils, oregano, kombu, and the stock. Bring the entire mixture to a boil, and reduce heat to a steady simmer. Cook until the lentils are nice and tender (about 45 minutes). Stir in the kale, parsley and the rice and cook for an additional 8-10 minutes. Stir in a teaspoon of pesto just before serving.

8. Congee

1 cup Brown rice

5 cups stock

1" piece of Ginger, peeled and grated

½ teaspoon Turmeric

¼ teaspoon Cayenne Pepper

½ teaspoon Coriander

Fresh sliced ginger

Sesame oil

Coriander (cilantro)

Green onions

Cayenne pepper

Ground turmeric

Place the ginger, turmeric, cayenne pepper and coriander in a greased pot and toast over a medium heat until aromatic. Add rice, stirring to coat with the spices. Pour the stock over and bring to a boil. Lower the heat to a simmer and slow cook for about an hour, making sure to stir regularly. It should look creamy when done. Spoon in the serving bowls and garnish with freshly sliced ginger, sesame oil, tamari, coriander, cayenne, and turmeric.

If you don't like brown rice, feel free to substitute quinoa, barley, or whole oats.

CHAPTER 6

Lunch or Dinner Recipes

While breakfasts for most people tend to be light, lunch and dinner meals usually require more substance. You still want it to be healthy and nutritious but you have to find ingredients that will boost the nutritional value of the food without adding in additional toxins or fats that will interfere with the immune system. These recipes will serve you well for that very purpose. You'll find that they are not only high in the nutrients, vitamins, and minerals your body needs, but they are also flavorful enough to keep you fully satisfied throughout the day.

1. Salmon Salad

2 cups of lettuce

¼ cup of carrots

¼ cup of onions

Vinegar

Seasonings (your preference)

3 ounces of poached salmon

Rice bread

Unsweetened berry juice

Combine lettuce, carrots, onions, vinegar, and the seasonings of your choice. Mix them together and dish them up on a plate. Serve with rice bread, and a cup of your favorite fresh berry juice.

2. Chicken Pasta

Olive oil

4 ounces of chicken breasts

¼ cup of marinara sauce

2 Tablespoons of breadcrumbs

Spaghetti

Heat olive oil in a saucepan and add in the chopped chicken breasts. Cook well. Add in the marinara sauce and top with breadcrumbs. Grill or broil until the breadcrumbs become brown. Serve over ½ cup of cooked spaghetti.

3. Crab Cakes

6 ounces of crabmeat

2 Tablespoons of egg whites

1 Tablespoon of your favorite seasonings

1 cup of broccoli

Mix the crabmeat, egg whites, and the seasonings together. Add oil to a skillet, add in the mixture and cook for 10 minutes. Serve over a bed of steamed broccoli.

4. Steak Salad

1 steak

2 cups of lettuce

Carrots

¼ cup of red onions

2 Tablespoons of champagne salad

Blue Cheese for garnish

Grill the steak to your liking. Mix lettuce, carrots, red onions, and champagne salad in a bowl. Add in a little Blue Cheese for a garnish and top it off with slices of grilled steak.

5. Beans Vinaigrette

2 pounds of cooked green beans

1 cup of diced red bell peppers

1 Tablespoon of unsweetened berry jam

2 Tablespoons of extra virgin olive oil

1 Tablespoon of white wine vinegar

1 teaspoon of Dijon mustard

1 teaspoon of coarse salt

¼ teaspoons of ground black pepper

Mix the cooked green beans, red bell peppers, and berry jam together. Mix in the extra virgin olive oil, white wine vinegar, Dijon mustard, salt and pepper together into a slightly thick sauce. Pour over the beans and toss to coat.

6. Turkey Chili

1 chopped onion

1 Tablespoon minced garlic

1 ½ pounds of ground turkey

2 cups of water

20 ounces of crushed or pureed tomatoes

2 Tablespoons of chili powder

2 teaspoons of turmeric

1 teaspoon of dried oregano

1 teaspoon of smoked paprika

1 teaspoon of cumin

Mix all the ingredients together in a large pot and bring to a boil. Reduce heat to a simmer and allow to cook for at least 45 minutes or until the flavors have all blended together.

7. Roasted Chicken with a Balsamic Vinaigrette

¼ cup of balsamic vinegar

2 Tablespoons of Dijon mustard

2 Tablespoons of lemon juice

2 chopped garlic cloves

2 Tablespoons of olive oil

Salt

Black pepper

4 lbs. of chicken, cut into pieces

½ cup of chicken broth

1 teaspoon of lemon zest

1 Tablespoon of fresh parsley, chopped

Mix the vinegar, mustard, lemon juice, garlic, olive oil, salt and pepper together in a bowl to make the vinaigrette. Pour the vinaigrette over the chicken and place it all in a sealable plastic bag. Seal and toss to coat the chicken. Refrigerate for at least 2 hours but no more than 1 day.

Preheat the oven to 400F. Remove the marinated chicken from the bag and spread out evenly in a large, prepared baking dish. Roast the chicken in the oven for about 1 hour. Transfer to a serving platter and place on a medium to low burner to keep warm.

Drain off the pan drippings and whisk together in a separate bowl, making sure to get the browned bits found on the bottom of the baking sheet and mix them in. Drizzle the mixture over the roasted chicken and sprinkle with lemon zest and parsley just before serving.

8. The Kitchen Sink

1 Tablespoon of grapeseed oil

Kosher salt

Black pepper

2 small yellow squash sliced into ½ in pieces

2 carrots (peeled and quartered)

1 medium chopped onion

2 Tablespoons of minced garlic

2 large potatoes, peeled and diced

2 quarts of vegetable stock

1 cup of navy beans (rinsed and drained)

Anti-Inflammatory Diet

1 cup of kidney beans (rinsed and drained)

1 bay leaf

2 teaspoons of minced thyme

2 cups of broccoli

2 medium chopped tomatoes (Roma)

Preheat the oven to 350F. In a mixing bowl mix together the grapeseed oil and the salt and pepper. Add in the squash, carrots, onion, garlic, and potatoes, and toss to make sure that they are coated completely. Place the tossed vegetables on a baking sheet and roast until the onions are tender and translucent. This should take about 20 to 30 minutes.

Place a large pot over medium heat, add the stock, beans, bay leaf, and the thyme. Cook for 10 minutes occasionally stirring. Put the stock mixture through a pulse blender until the beans are just beginning to puree. Remove the vegetables from the oven and add to the stock. Add the broccoli and tomatoes and stir until well mixed. Cook until all vegetables are thoroughly cooked, about another 30 minutes. Serve while still hot.

CHAPTER 7

Smoothies and Teas

Smoothies are a great way to get your nutrition without having to spend a lot of time in the kitchen. You can have a smoothie any time of the day or night but most people prefer them in the morning. They can also serve as a great snack when you get those hunger pangs in the middle of the day.

Other drinks also can be quite refreshing and relaxing. Teas have a lot of healing properties that will be very beneficial for boosting the immune system and fighting off that inflammation.

1. Raspberry Tea Smoothie

1½ cups of green tea

2 cups of fresh or frozen raspberries

1 banana

1 Tablespoon of honey

Place all the ingredients in a blender and mix until smooth. Add ice to chill and serve cold.

2. Rose Cranberry Tea

1 Tablespoon of rose hips

4 cups of water

¼ cup of cranberry juice

½ Tablespoon of stevia powder (optional)

Place all ingredients in a sauce pan and bring to a boil. Serve hot.

3. Ginger Tea

Add ginger root to your normal tea. This can also be done with nutmeg and cinnamon tea as well.

4. Green Ginger Smoothie

Watermelon

Ginger

Berries

Coconut water

Salt

Cayenne pepper

Place all the ingredients in a blender and blend until smooth. Serve cold.

5. Pear Apple Smoothie

½ pear

2/3 cup of diced pineapples

1 avocado

½ cucumber

½ teaspoon of dill

1 cup of spinach

1 stalk of celery

¼ teaspoon of turmeric

2 cups of water

Place all the ingredients in a blender and blend until smooth. Serve cold.

6. Green Ginger Smoothie

1 handful of baby spinach

1 inch of ginger, grated

1 clove of garlic

1 handful of watercress

1 avocado

½ a capsicum

1 cup of coconut water

Blend all the ingredients together until smooth. Add in a pinch of salt and cayenne pepper and blend again before serving.

These recipes are just a sample of what you can try for the first week of your anti-inflammatory diet. Once you've adapted to the type of foods that you can incorporate into your meals, you'll be able to adapt your normal recipes so that they fit within your anti-inflammatory diet plan. Keep reading to learn more about how to create new recipes, to increase the variety in your menus.

CHAPTER 8

Eat an Anti-Inflammatory Diet in Real Practice

This diet is not just for your reading pleasure. It needs to be incorporated into your regular eating routine and consistently followed over a period of weeks, months, or maybe even years. The recipes listed here are just the beginning. They should serve as a foundation for your new diet. If you stick to the regimen for long enough, you will see results, which should motivate you to seek out and try even more food options in the days and weeks to come.

You also need to keep in mind which foods to avoid while on the diet and recognize the triggers that may cause you to want to bounce back to your old habits. As you try these recipes and seek out new ones, try keeping a journal so you'll recognize the triggers that may make you falter and the driving forces that will help you to push forward for better results. Armed with this information, you'll be better prepared to make a success out of this new anti-inflammatory diet.

The Cheat Code

Of course, no one can start a diet completely from scratch and completely eliminate all the foods they love. It is likely going too far to ask you to quit your favorites cold turkey. So, imagine you are starting your diet today. Let's say that you forego all the foods that you love to eat and live on a diet of leafy vegetables, beetroots, spices, and other healthy foods. How long do you think you would survive on this diet? Chances are, it wouldn't be for very long. Your best option would be to take it step by step. To help you do this, use this cheat code.

- Whatever juice you make, add a few pieces of beetroot to it. A small amount of beetroot will not change the taste.
- Add a pinch of turmeric and other spices when you cook meat.
- Add flaxseed to all your smoothies and oatmeal recipes.
- If you are making pasta sauce, add a lot of flaxseeds and garlic to it.
- Add quinoa to your soup.

Anti-Inflammatory Diet

Add asparagus, cauliflower, and celery to your soup and wherever possible.

If you are planning to have a salad, add some smashed avocado to the dressing.

If you're a pizza lover, drizzle some flax oil, chia seeds and turmeric on the toppings. Serve the pizza with a side salad of tomato and avocado.

Following these simple cheats will help you to stay on the diet longer and the longer you stay on it, the easier it will be for it to become a habit, which will help you to make it more of a lifestyle change than a new novelty.

It will also help a great deal if you transition your new eating habits one at a time rather than jumping in all at once. By gradually easing yourself into the new diet, you give your body a chance to adjust to the new changes little by little. Try to incorporate each of the following steps into your diet one at a time to give you a better chance at success.

First, you need to cut back on caffeine. Reduce the number of cups of coffee that you consume per day. Also reduce the sugar content but do it slowly. If you're accustomed to adding two teaspoons of sugar to your cup, then cut down to 1 ½, then 1, then ½ and so on.

Have a timeline within which you should plan to incorporate the diet.

Start with one meal a day. By substituting one meal at a time you allow the body to get used to your new meal habit. Try

Anti-Inflammatory Diet

starting with something simple like snack foods to help you avoid snacking in between meals throughout the day. Once you've rid yourself of that habit you can move on to switching out each meal, one at a time.

Do not go for extracts or supplements if you can find fresh ingredients. For instance, if you can easily buy turmeric, do not substitute it with turmeric substitute pills. Whenever possible, go for the food source in its natural condition rather than factory made supplements.

Try to learn a lot of different recipes that will support your anti-inflammatory diet. This will keep the program interesting and your meal times exciting.

Do not stop any medications that you are presently taking to treat chronic inflammation. The effects of the anti-inflammatory diet might take time to show any considerable effects. If it is a serious inflammation problem you are dealing with such as lung inflammation (which could be life threatening) you'll want those medications to be working for you while the diet is taking effect. Do not substitute the medicine with the diet. As your inflammation improves, your doctor will start gradually easing your prescriptions. In the meantime, continue your medications as prescribed.

Do it as a group. Diets work best on the buddy system so find yourself a diet buddy to share the experience with. This way you will have a support system in place that will help you to stick with the diet for a longer period of time.

Remove seven inflammation prone foods from your diet each week. That's one food for each day. By eliminating these food choices one at a time it gives you a better chance at success.

Start by ridding your kitchen stock of all inflammatory foods. Stock it with simple snacks that do not violate the codes of the anti-inflammatory diet plan.

Try cheating on the diet every once in a while. Make it a diet free Friday or every other Friday. On your cheat day, you can consume all the foods you like but on Saturday morning you should get back to the anti-inflammatory diet in earnest once again. By allowing yourself a cheat day, you can reduce the stress that usually accompanies this type of dietary change.

Practical Restrictions

If you are vegan, you'll have to take up other protein substances to ensure that you get enough omega-3 fatty acids or you'll have to consume fish oil supplements. For those who are allergic to gluten, you should avoid consuming anything with wheat, barley, or rye. You can consume other grains such as quinoa and rice. Those who cannot consume salt should focus on eating more fruits and vegetables.

Whether your interest in the anti-inflammatory diet is because you're coping with a life threatening illness, or you simply want to manage your health better, it is strongly recommended that you seek the advice of a doctor before you proceed. Your doctor will be better able to gauge what parts of the diet will be more effective and which ones will need to be adjusted to meet your direct medical needs. This diet does not knowingly cause any interactions with drugs but some medical conditions might require that you add or remove certain foods that may be mentioned here in this book. Therefore, a doctor's advice is essential in those cases.

For anyone who is under 18 years of age, this diet might not be able to give the amount of calories that are needed for proper growth and development. So it is important to get in touch with your doctor to learn as much as you can about any additional foods that may need to be incorporated into your child's diet to ensure that he or she gets all the essential nutrients. The same applies for any mothers who are breastfeeding and pregnant women.

This chapter should act like a cheat code to help you to add as many anti-inflammatory items to your diet as possible without adding stress. This is important for a number of reasons. Stress is also an important cause of inflammation and many other problems that can affect your health. When you create more restrictions in your diet, you insert more pressure and stress into your system. So, to keep stress away, it is better to introduce this diet a little at a time, taking advantage of these stress codes to make sure that you ease your transition into your new eating habits.

CHAPTER 9

This Diet Can Still be Beneficial Even if Inflammation is Not a Problem

An anti-inflammatory diet is for those who have to deal with chronic inflammation and would like to take steps to reduce it through natural methods. But what about those who may not be dealing with chronic inflammation at all? Does this mean that there are no benefits to taking up this diet?

Keep reading to learn more about the other benefits you can get from this diet besides relieving you of excess inflammation.

This chapter is aimed at motivating you to continue this diet for as long as possible. There are a lot of diet plans that you may have followed in the past. Unlike those other diet plans, this anti-inflammatory diet does not provide you an assurance that you will lose 5 inches from your waist in a week or to get a bikini body for the beach season. But it does have its own set of advantages that can be of benefit to you.

If you are someone who does not have to contend with chronic inflammation or you are in a situation where you may be forced to take up this diet in support of a loved one, here are some practical points that can make you happy about trying this diet and bring you other benefits along with it.

Weight Reduction

The anti-inflammatory diet is not usually followed by those who want to lose weight but in the process of reducing inflammation and the pain it causes, you are also reducing your consumption of trans-fat, increasing the amount of proteins in your diet, and adding healthy fats to your body. These are all factors that can assist you in shedding those excess pounds you might want to get rid of.

In addition, as you consume more healthy proteins, and a lot more fruits and vegetables, it will naturally boost your weight loss.

Improves Joint Health

For those who have to cope with conditions like rheumatoid arthritis, this diet will help to reduce the pain and inflammation in your joints. It also helps in reducing morning stiffness and reduces the intensity of those painful episodes.

Improves Heart Health

All of the foods that you consume on this diet will help you to reduce your cholesterol levels, which will automatically improve the health of your heart. Moreover, this diet can also help you to get better control of your blood pressure levels, increase the amount of fiber in your diet, and help in reducing your CRP levels.

Diabetes

If you look at the type of foods you would be avoiding, you can easily understand that all the foods that would naturally spike your blood sugar levels are being eliminated. In fact, the foods you consume will actually encourage the body to produce more insulin, therefore it can be very beneficial for those who are suffering from diabetic problems or even those who are prone to this medical condition.

Liver Health

One of the first stages of liver disease is the inflammation of the liver. Before your liver is permanently damaged, this diet can help to cure any inflammation and slow down the onset of symptoms. An inflamed liver might be due to any number of conditions, including viral infection, which can also result in excess inflammation. This could lead to complications with the body's waste removal process. Other common factors that can lead to liver inflammation are drinking unclean water, not getting vaccinated for hepatitis A and B, poor personal hygiene or sexual hygiene, sharing needles or receiving bodily fluids from someone with hepatitis, and eating raw seafood. By coupling this diet with changing habits that could lead to inflammation of the liver, you can do wonders to improve your health.

Unlike other anti-inflammatory drugs and supplements, this diet does not mask or reduce the pain of inflammation alone. It works by addressing the root cause of the inflammation and helps to reduce its frequency in those who are prone to these kinds of health problems as a result of more severe medical conditions.

CONCLUSION

Thank you again for downloading this book!

I hope this book was able to help you to gain a better understanding of the anti-inflammatory diet and other tips for incorporating it into your life on a regular basis.

You may be someone who already knew about this diet, or you might be learning about it for the very first time. This book basically focuses on its practical uses for all kinds of readers. I hope you have gained a bit more insight about the diet plan and how it can benefit your health.

What to do next? It is not enough just to read the pages of this book. Even if you download hundreds of such books and learn all the contents by heart, it would be of no use to you unless you make practical application of it in your daily routine.

This book has dedicated a chapter to explaining to you the practical problems that you will face when you plan on taking up this diet. There are also a lot of tips provided for you to ease the transition into healthier eating habits. But keep in mind that each person is different. The way one person may react to a new diet plan is unpredictable and his or her responses will vary from others who take up the same diet. Use the tips, which have been provided in this book, and make sure to take up this diet one step at a time.

How long should you remain on this diet? You should know it is not some kind of medicine where you need to consume it for a considerable number of days and get the desired results. This diet will require a long and continuous process in order for it to be effective. While you might not be able to see the positive results within a very short period of time, the effect of this diet is certain and has been proven by a lot of scientific research. There are no side effects, which have been reported from those who are practicing this diet. Thus, all kinds of people can follow it.

Even if you find that you are not able to continue the diet and need to stop it before you see the results you seek, you'll find that there are a lot of people who have failed with other diets many times over but still have found success in the long run. It is important that you don't see your dropping the diet as a failure as this would cause you to lose hope even with the slightest slip. When you are ready, try again and take advantage of the cheat codes to help you get back on the right track. Introduce the program in smaller increments so that you'll have a better chance of success in the end. We wish you the best of success in your attempts to control your chronic inflammation and get better health as a result. By starting this diet and making it a part of your life, you are in fact, taking an active role in protecting your health and improving your quality of life at the same time.

The next step is entirely up to you. So go out there and take control of your life and reclaim your health but starting your own anti-inflammatory diet plan.

Finally, if you enjoyed this book, then I'd like to ask you for a favor, would you be kind enough to leave a review for this book on Amazon? It'd be greatly appreciated!

Thank you and good luck!

CHECK OUT MY OTHER BOOKS

Below you'll find some of my other popular books that are popular on Amazon and Kindle as well. Simply click on the links below to check them out. Alternatively, you can visit my author page on Amazon to see other work done by me.

If the links do not work, for whatever reason, you can simply search for these titles on the Amazon website to find them.

BOOKS BY LR SMITH:

Low Carb High Fat - Click here

Ketogenic Diet - Click here

Mediterranean Diet - Click here

Whole Food - Click here

Dash Diet - Click here

Bone Broth - Click here

Printed in Great Britain
by Amazon